Fit For The Kingdom
Eat, Pray, Train

K.D. Roland

ISBN-13: 978-1720361480
ISBN-10: 1720361487

I dedicate this book to my lord and savior, Jesus Christ. He has showered me with unconditional love, forgiveness, and blessings. I am forever grateful for this beautiful life I've been given.

Contents:

Introduction

Welcome to Fit for the Kingdom! Thank you for purchasing this book and deciding to grow in your faith and fitness! I hope you are encouraged by the words you find on these pages, are challenged by the workouts, and are delighted with the recipes. You can consider this a 4-week transformation program!

You may think of Fit for the Kingdom in one of two ways: present or future. You can use this book as a tool to help you improve your health and mindset for the here and now. The workouts will challenge you physically and the scripture verses will challenge you spiritually. As you strengthen your relationship with your creator and tap into the resources He has given you, you will be "Fit for the Kingdom." You will be healthier and more grounded and can invest in others or "pay it forward."

You can also use this book as a tool to get you excited about what is to come. We know that our time here on earth is only temporary. When we pass through death and into eternity, we will arrive at God's kingdom! The scripture verses in this book are meant for encouragement and to remind you who you are and where you are going. You will be reminded to place your focus on heavenly things, to fear less, and trust more.

Each verse will have a few questions following it. Take some time to think about the verse and answer the questions. There is space for you to record your thoughts. The verses have been taken from the NIV version of the Bible. As you know, the mind is a powerful tool and can be used for us or against us. You will see the command to "renew your mind" often times throughout scripture!

In the "getting started" section you have ways to monitor your progress. Write down your base information and take note along the way. When I am training clients, I measure weight weekly and inches monthly. I also test their strength and endurance with exercises such as: 1 mile walk or jog, holding a plank, and a max bench press or squat.

People get motivated to continue when they see the positive changes the routine is having on their bodies and lives! Please remember, working out is not always about losing weight. You will gain several other benefits such as: improved posture and flexibility, lowered blood pressure and cholesterol, as well as, added years to your life!

Please consult your physician before beginning the workout routine. Always stop the exercise if you have pain. Take your time and do a slow, controlled movement. The workouts gradually get more challenging. The first week is composed of basic exercises to strengthen upper body, lower body, and core. They are set up as a split routine to avoid total body soreness. The next three weeks will build upon the first week. You will try different set and rep counts, challenge your balance and stability, and hopefully lift more weight! To see a video of each exercise, please visit my YouTube site- Danielle Roland, CPT.

I suggest taking note of the weight you use as well as the number of reps and sets you complete of each exercise. Over time, you will see that you can lift more and do more! You can also repeat a workout week if you are not ready to move forward. The beauty of these workouts is they don't expire! Enjoy them, have fun, and always challenge yourself!

Near the back of the book you will find several of my favorite recipes. I have included the source as they are not my own. You may also find other recipes that interest you as you browse the websites! A few other nutrition tips would be to: drink plenty of water, eat 3-4 times a day, track your calories and macros, and eat out less.

Getting Started- Tools for Tracking Progress

Measurements (in inches)

Shoulders-

Chest-

Bicep-

Abdominals-

Hips-

Thigh-

Calf-

Body composition

Weight-

Body fat %-

Strength and endurance (time or lbs)

Plank hold-

Bench press max-

Squat/Leg press max-

1 mile-

Week 1

"The thief comes only to steal and kill and destroy; I have come that they may have life, and have it to the full." (John 10:10, New International Version)

1. Who is the thief?
2. Who comes to give life?
3. What do you consider a "full" life?

Reflect:

____
____
____
____
____
____
____
____
____
____
____
____
____
____
____
____
____
____
____
____
____
____

Today's workout focuses on your upper body. We will do some of the basic exercises to gain strength and muscle tone. To create symmetry and avoid injury you should always train opposite muscle groups equally. For example, here you will see that you train your biceps and then your triceps or your back and then your chest.

Upper Body Workout:

Equipment needed- dumbbells, bench or swiss ball
Complete 3 sets of 15 reps each exercise
For demo of exercises: YouTube- Danielle Roland, CPT

1. Standing bicep curl

2. Seated overhead tricep extension

3. Front and lateral deltoid raise

4. Chest press (on bench or swiss ball)

5. Bent over row

Cardio- 30 minutes of light to moderate activity

Notes:

____

____

____

____

____

____

"Therefore, if anyone is in Christ, the new creation has come: The old has gone, the new is here!" (2 Corinthians 5:17, New International Version)

1. What does it mean to be "in Christ?"
2. How do you become a new creation?
3. Have you become a new creation? If so, how have you changed most?

Reflect:

Today's workout focuses on your lower body. The exercises work several muscles at once. When performing these exercises be careful that you do not experience back pain. Keep alignment of the hips, knees, and ankles.

Lower Body Workout

Equipment needed: dumbbell / barbell, resistance band or cable machine
Complete 3 sets of 15 reps each exercise
For demo of exercises- YouTube- Danielle Roland, CPT

1. Alternating lunge

2. Single leg bridge

3. Squat

4. Deadlift (hold 2 dumbbells or barbell)

5. 4-way leg raise (with resistance band or cable)

Cardio- 30 minutes of light to moderate activity

Notes-

____
____
____
____
____

"For physical training is of some value, but godliness has value for all things, holding promise for both the present life and the life to come." (1 Timothy 4:8, New International Version)

1. Name some examples of physical training?
2. How does someone become "godly."
3. Name some examples of "godly" training.

Reflect:

____
____
____
____
____
____
____
____
____
____
____
____
____
____
____
____
____
____
____
____
____
____
____

Today's workout focuses on your core. Your core is also known as your trunk or your "powerhouse." It is also the place where balance starts. During core exercises, keep your abdominals tight and engaged. Do not allow your back to arch when performing exercises on the floor.

Core workout

Equipment needed: medicine ball
Complete 3 sets of 15 reps each exercise
For demo of exercises- YouTube- Danielle Roland, CPT

1. Bird dog

2. Dead bug

3. Pike

4. Russian twist (use medicine ball)

5. Plank mountain climber

Cardio- 30 minutes of light to moderate activity

Notes:

____
____
____
____
____

Week 2

"not giving up meeting together, as some are in the habit of doing, but encouraging one another and all the more as you see the day approaching." (Hebrews 10:25, New International Version)

1. What type of meeting is this verse referring to?
2. Explain how other believers encourage you.
3. Why do you need accountability in both fitness and faith?

Reflect:
____
____
____
____
____
____
____
____
____
____
____
____
____
____
____
____
____
____
____
____
____
____
____
____

Today's workout will combine the exercises you learned last week to make the routine a bit more functional and advanced. You will be performing movements that are useful in everyday activities. Take your time and pay close attention to form.

Full Body Workout

Equipment needed: dumbbells, bench
Complete 4 sets of 10 reps of each exercise as a circuit
For demo of exercises- YouTube- Danielle Roland, CPT

1. Walking lunge with bicep curl

2. Squat to shoulder press

3. Renegade row

4. Chest press with leg raise

5. Tricep dip

Cardio- 30 minutes of interval training

Notes:

____
____
____
____
____
____

"Have I not commanded you? Be strong and courageous. Do not be afraid; do not be discouraged, for the Lord your God will be with you wherever you go." (Joshua 1:9, New International Version)

1. Have you ever been courageous? Describe the situation.
2. How has fear limited you in your life?
3. Do you believe that God will be with you in everything?

Reflect:

Today's workout is primarily body weight training. Try to increase the intensity of your workout and push yourself! As you will see, you don't have to lift heavy weights to get a great workout.

Full Body Workout

Equipment needed: medicine ball
Complete 4 sets of 10 reps of each exercise as a circuit
For demo of exercises- YouTube- Danielle Roland, CPT

1. Wall ball

2. Burpee

3. Side plank hip tap

4. Bicycle crunch

5. Push up

Cardio- 30 minutes of interval training

Notes:

____
____
____
____
____
____
____

"Before I formed you in the womb I knew you, before you were born I set you apart; I appointed you as a prophet to the nations." (Jeremiah 1:5, New International Version)

1. How does it feel knowing you have a creator?
2. What does it mean to be "set apart?"
3. What gifts and talents has God given you that may help build the kingdom?

Reflect:

____
____
____
____
____
____
____
____
____
____
____
____
____
____
____
____
____
____
____
____
____
____

Today's workout is all about the kettlebell! The kettlebell is great because you can use one device to gain cardio and strength training! You can hit all muscle groups and create fun, interesting workouts. While using the kettlebell, try and keep your motions fluid and continuous.

Kettlebell Workout

Equipment needed: kettlebell
Complete 4 sets of 10 reps of each exercise as a circuit
For demo of exercises- YouTube- Danielle Roland, CPT

1. Swing

2. Deadlift

3. Figure 8

4. Lunge and pass through

5. Turkish get up

Cardio- 30 minutes of interval training

Notes:

____
____
____
____
____

Week 3

"Since, then, you have been raised with Christ, set your hearts on things above, where Christ is, seated at the right hand of God. Set your minds on things above, not on earthly things. For you died, and your life is now hidden with Christ in God." (Colossians 3:1-3, New International Version)

1. How do you become "raised with Christ?"
2. What does it mean to set your heart on something?
3. Compare and contrast things that are above with earthly things.

Reflect:

____
____
____
____
____
____
____
____
____
____
____
____
____
____
____
____
____
____
____
____

Today's workout will be set up like a pyramid. This type of workout allows you to increase your weight without compromising your form. Bodybuilders will often use this style of workout to push their muscles to failure. The look of a bodybuilder may not be what you are going for but it is still a good way to see what you can do!

Upper Body Workout

Equipment needed: dumbbells, cable machine, bench
Complete 3 sets of 10, 8, 6 reps. Add weight each set
For demo of exercises- YouTube- Danielle Roland, CPT

1. Concentration curl

2. Standing tricep extension (on cable machine)

3. Seated shoulder press

4. Bench press

5. Seated row

Cardio- 45 minutes of moderate activity

Notes:

____
____
____
____
____
____

"So whether you eat or drink or whatever you do, do it all for the glory of God." (1 Corinthians 10:31, New International Version)

1. How do you bring glory to God?
2. Why does God deserve to be glorified?
3. How can you point others to Jesus through your profession and/or hobbies?

Reflect:

Today's workout places emphasis on gaining hip mobility. Did you know that over 15 muscles work together to provide movement at the hip joint? Athletes rely heavily on these muscles to perform actions such as: running, jumping, swimming, etc. Mobility in your hips also decreases back pain!

Lower Body Workout

Equipment needed: bench, dumbbells
Complete 2 sets of 20 each exercise
For demo of exercises- YouTube- Danielle Roland, CPT

1. Step up with knee drive

2. Goblet squat

3. Single leg deadlift

4. Fire hydrant

5. Plie squat

Cardio- 45 minutes of moderate activity

Notes:

____
____
____
____
____
____
____

"I can do all this through him who gives me strength."
(Philippians 4:13, New International Version)

1. When is the last time you felt weak?
2. Describe a situation that you overcame that seemed impossible.
3. Do you pray for strength during difficult times?

Reflect:

Today's workout is with the use of a swiss ball. You may also hear it called the "stability ball." It is great for strengthening your core as well as increasing balance. People also use it as a chair in offices or at home for postural reinforcement.

Swiss Ball Workout

Equipment needed: swiss ball
Complete 2 sets of 20 reps of each exercise
For demo of exercises- YouTube- Danielle Roland, CPT

1. Hand/feet pass off

2. Crunch

3. Scissor lift

4. Trunk rotation (supine)

5. Knee tuck

Cardio- 45 minutes of moderate activity

Notes:

____
____
____
____
____
____
____

Week 4

"For God so loved the world that he gave his one and only Son, that whoever believes in him shall not perish but have eternal life." (John 3:16, New International Version)

1. How does God show His love for the world?
2. According to this verse, how do you receive eternal life?
3. Have you placed faith in Jesus as your savior?

Reflect:

Today's workout is boxing and kickboxing! We all need to release a little tension at times! This workout may be new to you but with a little practice, you will get the hang of it! Boxing is great for total body conditioning. Always keep your abdominals engaged and have soft joints. No equipment needed!

Full Body Workout

For demo of exercises- YouTube- Danielle Roland, CPT

1. Reverse lunge and kick 3x15 each side

2. Cross punch 3x50

3. Side-kick 3x15 each side

4. Upper-cut 3x50

5. Squat jump 2x15

Cardio- 60 minutes of moderate activity

Notes:

____
____
____
____
____
____

"Gracious words are a honeycomb, sweet to the soul and healing to the bones." (Proverbs 16:24, New International Version)

1. What does it mean to be gracious?
2. How do words destroy others? How do words build others up?
3. Do you speak kind words to yourself? About yourself?

Reflect:

Today's workout will be focused on using the BOSU. It can be used on both sides for training balance, strength, and endurance. As you will see in this workout, there are several exercises that you can perform with it. If you don't already own one, I would add it to your list!

BOSU Workout

Equipment needed: Bosu
For demo of exercises- YouTube- Danielle Roland, CPT

1. Alternating lunge 2x20

2. Plank mountain climber 2x30

3. Push up 2x15

4. Squat 2x15

5. Up and overs 2x30

Cardio- 60 minutes of moderate activity

Notes:

____

____

____

____

____

____

____

"Yet to all who did receive him, to those who believed in his name, he gave the right to become children of God." (John 1:12, New International Version)

1. Name the most thoughtful gift you have ever received.
2. What does it mean to believe in the name of Jesus?
3. Are you a child of God? How does that make you feel?

Reflect:

Today's workout is with the use of the TRX. This device incorporates body weight training and really challenges your core. I love the TRX because you can take it with you anywhere! I have used this piece of equipment with almost all of my clients.

TRX Workout

Equipment needed: TRX
Complete 3 sets of 15 each exercise
For demo of exercises- YouTube- Danielle Roland, CPT

1. Chest press

2. High row

3. Pistol squat

4. Running man

5. Plank

Cardio- 60 minutes of moderate activity

Notes:

____

____

____

____

____

Congratulations, you finished the 30 day challenge! How do you feel? I truly enjoyed sharing my favorite verses, workouts, and recipes with you. I hope that you learned something new and will share it with others.

Don't forget to take your measurements and compare them to your baseline data! I know you will be shocked at your progress! You can pat yourself on the back because you truly put in the work!

As you move on from this study, continue to grow in your faith and fitness. You may decide to join K.D.'s virtual training for further training and accountability! Continue to challenge yourself and practice the habits you learned in this study. You will feel better and look better with each new day!

Recipes

Breakfast:

Quinoa Breakfast Scramble
https://wendypolisi.com/quinoa-breakfast-scramble/

Skinny Pumpkin Quinoa Muffins
https://www.simplyquinoa.com/skinny-pumpkin-quinoa-muffins/

Vanilla Almond Overnight Oats
https://realhousemoms.com/vanilla-almond-overnight-oats/

Berry Acai Bowl
http://leangreennutritionfiend.com/berry-acai-bowl/

Healthy Kale Egg Breakfast Cups
https://tasteandsee.com/healthy-kale-egg-breakfast-cups

Banana Oat Breakfast Smoothie
http://www.runningwithspoons.com/2016/05/03/banana-oat-breakfast-smoothie/

Key Lime Pie Protein Smoothie
https://www.theseasonedmom.com/key-lime-pie-protein-smoothie/

Lunch:

Loaded Guacamole Vegetarian Tacos
https://soupaddict.com/2014/06/loaded-guacamole-vegetarian-tacos/

Mediterranean Quinoa Salad
https://www.theharvestkitchen.com/mediterranean-quinoa-salad

Cheeseburger Lettuce Wraps
https://life-in-the-lofthouse.com/cheeseburger-lettuce-wraps/

Greek Yogurt Egg Salad Sandwich
https://damndelicious.net/2013/02/17/greek-yogurt-egg-salad-sandwich-sundaysupper/

Mediterranean Salad
http://cleanfoodcrush.com/mediterranean-salad/

Steak Fajita Burrito Bowl
https://www.joyfulhealthyeats.com/steak-fajita-burrito-bowls/

BLT Chicken Salad Stuffed Avocados
http://www.thegarlicdiaries.com/blt-chicken-salad-stuffed-avocados/

Mexican Kale Salad
https://ifoodreal.com/mexican-kale-salad/

Avocado Lime Dressing
https://www.runninginaskirt.com/healthy-creamy-avocado-lime-dressing/2/

Dinner:

Italian Sausage and Brown Rice Stuffed Acorn Squash
https://thebusybaker.ca/stuffed-acorn-squash/

Slow Cooker Buffalo Chicken Stuffed Sweet Potato
https://therealfoodrds.com/slow-cooker-buffalo-chicken/

Low Carb Cauliflower Pot Pies
http://www.itscheatdayeveryday.com/low-carb-cauliflower-pot-pies/

Sausage Stuffed Portobello Mushrooms
https://www.foxandbriar.com/sausage-stuffed-portobello-mushrooms/

Cilantro Lime Black Bean Burgers
https://www.lemonsandzest.com/2015/06/17/cilantro-lime-black-bean-burgers/

Baked Eggplant with lentils, tomatoes, and herby topping
https://quitegoodfood.co.nz/baked-eggplant-lentils-tomatoes-herby-topping/

Spicy Shrimp Cauliflower Mash Roasted Kale
https://pinchofyum.com/spicy-shrimp-cauliflower-mash-roasted-kale

Chicken Pesto Kabobs
https://damndelicious.net/2016/06/04/chicken-pesto-kabobs/

Snacks:

Cinnamon Apple Chips
https://www.carriesexperimentalkitchen.com/cinnamon-apple-chips/

Matcha No Bake Energy Bites
https://theloopywhisk.com/2017/07/31/matcha-no-bake-energy-bites-video/

Cranberry Almond Granola Bars
http://www.leancleanandbrie.com/2017/02/cranberry-almond-granola-bars.html

Mexican Chocolate Avocado Ice Cream
https://alldayidreamaboutfood.com/low-carb-mexican-chocolate-avocado-ice-cream/

Ultimate Paleo Trail Mix
http://nurturemygut.com/ultimate-paleo-trail-mix.html/

Clean Eating Spinach Artichoke Dip
http://meaningfuleats.com/clean-eating-spinach-artichoke-dip-dairy-free/

Homemade Beef Jerky
https://thegirlonbloor.com/recipe-homemade-beef-jerky/

Biography

K.D. Roland is originally from West Virginia. She grew up in Florida and currently resides in the Tampa Bay area. She loves the outdoors, loves to travel, and competes in road races and triathlons. Her 7 year old labrador, Champ, keeps her on the go at all times!

She received her bachelor's degree in athletic training from the University of South Florida and her master's degree in counseling from Southeastern Baptist Theological Seminary. K.D. has worked in various settings using both skills including: NC State University, St. David's School, Florida Orthopedic Institute, and D1 Sports Training.

With experience in a wide range of settings, she decided to start her own personal training business in 2015. FemaleF.I.R.S.T, Inc. was originally developed to properly condition female high school and college athletes to avoid debilitating injury. The program would be: Functional, Individualized, Resistive, Sport-specific, and Total body. She has had great success working with athletes. The difference lies in how you train.

Over the past 3 years, K.D. had expanded her client base to men and women between the ages of 16-70. She has trained people of all walks of life with various types of goals. She also offers virtual training. You can get everything she offers her one-on-one clients remotely! Virtual training has given her the opportunity to reach more people.

Fit For The Kingdom is her way of combining both of her passions: fitness and faith. K.D. decided to write this book to encourage people to get in their best health and discover their true worth. She simply wants to remind you that greater things lie ahead!

Fit for the Kingdom will be at least 3 volumes. She plans to release volume 2 during the Fall of 2018. Each volume will offer words of encouragement, recipes, and different fitness routines. Stay tuned for another 4 week transformation!

K.D. Roland is active on social media. You can find her on Instagram as Lipstiknlunges and Facebook as FemaleFirst, Inc. Please check out her pages and follow along!

You may also visit her website to gain more information about the business, join her monthly e-newsletter, or inquire about virtual training at www.femalefirst1.com

www.ingramcontent.com/pod-product-compliance
Lightning Source LLC
Chambersburg PA
CBHW070101260726
48658CB00002B/937